W0115579

THE
COOKIE
JOURNAL

Shay Pcok

The Cookie Journal
© Shay Pcok

ISBN: 978-1-66786-895-0

HEALTH LITERACY IS VITAL.

Our book series were created with all women and men in mind who just may have questions and concerns about womb health and prostate issues. And for those who personally do not have current issues or concerns when it comes to your womanly anatomy, or your manly parts, we're positive that you'll still find the contents of the book series titled, The Cookie Journal enlightening, educational and quite informative, and for those who are currently experiencing some sort of dreadful side effect/s related to the matters of womb or prostate life, you'll find we have come up with several natural remedies with you in mind, and lastly for those who just may know of someone who perhaps are continuously experiencing the downslope of dealing with reoccurrence of womb issues or negligent prostate maintenance, you'll find this book widely knowledgeable for you to the point that you'll be able to do more that just give that first mind advice paraphrase, "go see a doctor" love one/friend, you'll be so adeptly equipped that you'll be able to suggest valuable treasured natural help right away, right from the top of your head, without a second guess, you'll also be ready and capable to answer the questions of your love one/friend that is dealing with the issue/s. The Cookie Journal book series is here to succinctly cover all the salient points of proper womb care and proper prostate maintenance.

KNOWING THE DIFFERENCE

Now if you find yourself saying, it itches, it burns, it's painful and swollen.

What is it? Where did it come from? What can I do to rid myself of it?

"I know something is seriously wrong with me" I just saw my doctor for the exact same symptoms a month ago.

Have you ever found yourself wondering and asking yourself any of the mentioned questions above?

Knowing the warning signs the preventive measures and the proper diagnosis can certainly help you to prevent reoccurring urinary tract infections, bacteria vaginosis and yeast infections.

Knowing the difference between yeast infection, urinary tract infection and bacteria vaginosis.

VAGINAL YEAST INFECTION

is a fungal infection that causes irritation, discharge and intense itchiness of the vagina and the vulva — the tissues at the vaginal opening.

Also called vaginal candidiasis, vaginal yeast infection affects up to 3 out of 4 women at some point in their lifetimes.

SYMPTOMS

Requires medical diagnosis

Yeast infection symptoms can range from mild to moderate, and include:

- Itching and irritation in the vagina and vulva
- A burning sensation, especially during intercourse or while urinating
- Redness and swelling of the vulva
- Vaginal pain and soreness
- Vaginal rash

- Thick, white, odor-free vaginal discharge with a cottage cheese appearance

KEY POINT

A vaginal yeast infection isn't considered a sexually transmitted infection. But, there's an increased risk of vaginal yeast infection at the time of first regular sexual activity. There's also some evidence that infections may be linked to mouth to genital contact (oral-genital sex).

TREATMENT

Prescribed medication/s can effectively treat vaginal yeast infections. If you suffer with reoccurring yeast infections — four or more within a year — you may need a longer treatment course and a maintenance plan.

Did you know once diagnosed and treated by a medical doctor, you can avoid future reoccurring yeast infections all simply by practicing the age old remedy Yoni Steaming with herbs.

This practice has been used for centuries in the African culture and West Indies and have since grown in recent popularity. Yoni Steaming with Herbs is done simply by the use of a natural herbs. That's right all natural.

We will get more into steaming with herbs farther along.

KEY POINT

Bacteria Vaginosis

Bacterial overgrowth in the vagina.

Bacterial vaginosis tends to affect women of childbearing age. Activities that change the balance of bacteria in the vagina, such as sexual intercourse or frequent douching, can increase a person's risk.

SYMPTOMS

Requires medical diagnosis

In some cases, there are no symptoms. In other cases, there may be

- abnormal vaginal discharge, itching, or odor.

TREATMENT

Prescribed cream, gel, or oral medication. Reoccurring within three to 12 months is common, requiring additional treatment.

You can avoid future reoccurring bacteria vaginosis all simply by practicing the age old remedy Yoni Steaming with herbs.

MEN AND YEAST INFECTIONS

Can a man also get a yeast infection? Yes males sure can, which when they have yeast infection and it goes untreated it can lead to a condition known as balanitis which is inflammation at the head of the penis. Yeast Infection in males are common because the fungus that causes yeast infections(candida) is usually present on skin, especially moist skin. Balanitis is actually more common in uncircumcised men.

SIGNS AND SYMPTOMS

Moist skin on the penis, possibly with areas of a thick white substance collecting in folds.

- Area of shiny white skin

- Redness itching and burning sensation on the penis
- Higher Risk
- Aren't circumcised
- Use of antibiotics for prolonged periods
- Have diabetes
- Have an impaired immune system such as with HIV
- Are overweight
- Practice poor hygiene
- Treatment

Most males are treated with over the counter anti fungal medications

KEY POINT

- Urinary Tract Infection/ UTI
- An infection in any part of the urinary system, the kidneys, bladder, or urethra.
- Urinary tract infections are more common in women. They usually occur in the bladder or urethra, but more serious infections involve the kidney.

SYMPTOMS

Usually self diagnose however lab test to determine.

A bladder infection may cause pelvic pain, increased urge to urinate, pain with urination, and blood in the urine. A kidney infection may cause back pain, nausea, vomiting, and fever.

TREATMENT

Common treatment is with antibiotics.

So now that we've discussed 3 of the most common bacteria infections that women can encounter, that are not a sexual transmitted disease. Let's talk about steaming with herbs and it's beneficial components. Steaming with herbs traces back for centuries, where the women in other countries would use this form of remedy for cleansing and healing themselves naturally. Whereas traveling to and from local doctors due to limited village access and the distance to travel by bus or foot to obtain health care was extreme. The village women had always known about all natural herbs and their amazing powers, healing components and positive effects so they decided to test the theory out on themselves using boiling water and a mixture of these natural herbs. Unbeknownst to the village women who'd recently given birth, it reduced their recovery time significantly, also various village women who suffered with womb irritation and foul odors and irregular menses, it had begun to work wonders for them also. Boiling water combined with an assortment of natural herbs had become the local village women way of assisting themselves with their various womb issues. The village women began steaming with all natural herbs for self care.

PH BALANCING

The term 'pH' stands for 'potential of hydrogen,' which is the measure of a solution's hydrogen ion concentration. It is a measure of acidity or alkalinity on a scale of 0 to 14 – Zero being extremely acidic, 14 being extremely alkaline and 7 being neutral. When a solution is neutral it means there is complete balance between acid and alkaline. The human body tries to keep a tight range around neutral on the pH scale – between 6.8 (slightly acidic) and 7.4 (slightly alkaline). The most important thing to remember is that your blood pH needs to be maintained between 7.365 and 7.400. This is because blood needs to be slightly alkaline to nourish your tissues, organs and organ systems.

The foods you eat, the liquids you drink, your environment, your breathing patterns, and your exercise routine (or lack thereof) all have the potential to increase acidity in the body and negatively affect your blood pH. This happens because your body stores excess acid in your tissues which creates a more acidic body pH. To bring your body back into balance, your blood needs to pull from alkaline stores in your body – such as water, calcium, magnesium and potassium. To give you an example, the phosphoric acid in soda has a pH of 2.8. It is estimated to take roughly 32 glasses of pure water to neutralize the effects of one glass of soda!

All of your detoxification organs and systems – liver, kidneys, intestines, lungs and lymphatic system – help your body balance its pH. Of these, your kidneys are the major pH balancer. But if there is excess acidity that your kidneys can't handle, bones and muscles can also suffer. If the body becomes overly acidic, calcium is withdrawn from your bones to neutralize that acidity. This can eventually weaken bones and lead to osteoporosis. Additionally, excessive acidity can pull glutamine from skeletal muscle to help restore the body's pH. This can lead to difficulty gaining or even maintaining muscle mass.

If your diet, environment and lifestyle constantly keep your blood pH imbalanced, even a little bit, your body loses its effectiveness at neutralizing and eliminating those acid waste products from your system. This creates a chronic state of acidity in the tissues, increasing your risk of disease.

ACID-ALKALINE IMBALANCE

Common early signs of acid-alkaline imbalance include: allergies, breathing disorders, chronic colds and flus, headaches, indigestion, inflammation, fatigue, muscle cramping, pain, skin troubles and sinus problems. As acid continues to accumulate in the body, several organs and glands become effected including your thyroid, adrenal glands and liver. This can lead to many other health conditions. In fact, research has linked the following diseases and conditions to an underlying pH imbalance:

- Allergies
- Alzheimer's disease
- Arteriosclerosis
- Arthritis
- Bone fractures
- Bronchitis
- Cancer
- Candida overgrowth
- Cardiovascular disease
- Chronic fatigue syndrome
- Chronic infections
- Dementia
- Depression
- Diabetes
- Fibromyalgia
- Heart attacks

- High blood pressure
- High cholesterol
- Hormonal imbalances
- Immune deficiencies
- Insulin sensitivity
- Kidney disease
- Lou Gehrig's disease
- Multiple sclerosis
- Muscular dystrophy
- Obesity
- Osteoarthritis
- Osteoporosis
- Parkinson's disease
- Premature aging
- Premature hair graying
- Prostate problems
- Senility
- Sinusitis
- Stroke
- Tooth decay and loss of teeth
- Weight problems

If you have any of the following conditions above, you may have an acid-alkaline imbalance.

CAUSES OF ACID-ALKALINE IMBALANCE

There are several lifestyle and nutrition choices that could be increasing acidity in your body. Here are the top five categories:

- Stress. If your body is frequently in 'fight or flight' mode, your body is constantly secreting stress hormones. This not only creates inflammation in the body, it also increases acidity.

- Shallow breathing. Chronic stress also leads to rapid and shallow breathing or even holding your breath. Oxygen alkalizes your blood so reduced oxygen intake from this type of breathing pattern can increase acidity in the body.

- Toxins. Pesticides and other chemicals in conventional produce and meats; heavy metals; industrial pollutants; hormones and other chemicals found in foods, plastics, cleaning supplies and beauty products; and even potential chemicals in your tap water all increase acidity in the body.

- Infections. Infections create a more acidic environment which, in turn, makes you more vulnerable to germs leading to a vicious cycle.

- Acidic Diet. Sugar, refined flours, food additives, table salt, trans fats, fried foods, meat, dairy, alcohol and caffeine make it difficult for your body to restore its pH balance.

GET BACK INTO PH BALANCE

Use the following tips to decrease acidity in your body, reduce risk of diseases and optimize health.

- Reduce or Eliminate harmful acidic foods from your diet. Sugar. Sugar not only throws your pH levels out of balance, but excessive sugar consumption creates the perfect environment for overgrowth of yeast, fungi and pathogenic bacteria which can compromise health. Refined Flours. White flour, all baked goods made from refined flours (including some "multigrain" and "wheat" breads), and white rice are acid-forming in the body. Food Additives. Artificial flavors, colors, sweeteners and preservatives are not only acid-forming in the body, but many also have neurotoxic effects. Table Salt. Your average table salt is acid-forming. However, the good news is that sea salt, especially Celtic and Himalayan, are alkalizing on the body. This is because they contain an alkalizing form of sodium as well as other minerals like potassium and calcium which help combat acidity in the body. Unhealthy Fats. Trans fats and rancid fats from fried foods are both acid-forming in the body. Processed Foods. Packaged and processed fast foods have most if not all of the ingredients above - sugar, refined flour, food additives, salt, and unhealthy fats. Meats and Dairy. Almost all animal products are highly acid-forming, including beef, veal, pork, bacon, luncheon meats, eggs, milk, cheese, organ meats, poultry, farm-raised fish and shellfish. Cutting back on your consumption of these foods, and switching to organic, grass-fed, free range options will make it easier to balance your pH. Alcohol.

Alcohol is highly acid-forming in the body. In addition to alcohol's high sugar content, the ethanol in alcohol converts to acetaldehyde, a toxic by-product that also occurs in car emissions, tobacco smoke and industrial processes. Caffeine. Excessive caffeine consumption can increase acidity in the body. Certain Fruits, Vegetables and Nuts. Canned fruit, fruit syrups, fruit juices, jams, jellies, mushrooms, white potatoes, and salted nuts all increase acidity in the body. Choose healthier acidic foods. Having a 100% alkaline diet is not healthy either. Again, it's about balance. So choose healthier options for acidic foods and keep them at a low level in your diet – approximately 30%. Choose organic, grass-fed, free range and wild caught for meats, poultry and fish.Fresh Fruits. Yes, fruits can be acidic in the body. But they are full of fiber, vitamins, antioxidants and phytonutrients so they should still be a part of a whole foods diet. Just limit your consumption to fresh, organic fruits and eat more veggies than fruit. Black beans, kidney beans and chickpeas. Again, although these specific beans may be more acidic, they are still a good option for your whole food meal plan. Oats, brown rice, wild rice, amaranth and millet. All grains are acidic, but these are less acidic than wheat and refined flour's. Raw, unsalted nuts and seeds. Cold-pressed and/or virgin oils. Honey and maple syrup. These are still sugars, but can be part of an alkalizing diet in small quantities. Increase alkaline foods to 70% of your diet. All vegetables. Especially when organic and raw, veggies are very alkalizing. Yams, sweet potatoes, turnips, rutabaga, jicama, taro root, onion, kohlrabi, parsnips, beets and other root crops. These help quickly alkalize the body. Legumes. Organic soybeans, lentils, and lima beans help reduce acidity in the body. Avocados, coconut, lemon, lime, grapefruit, tomatoes and sour cherries. These fruits (yes avocados and tomatoes are fruits!) are very alkalizing to the body. Buckwheat groats and quinoa. These "grains" are not really grains at all, but seeds. They not only have complete proteins but also help reduce acidity. Almonds, pumpkin seeds, sesame seeds and sprouted seeds. Almonds and almond milk are very alkaline as are sprouted seeds. Avocado oil, coconut oil, flaxseed oil, olive oil and fish oil. Healthy oils can be a part of an alkalizing diet. Peppermint tea, yerba mate tea and lemon water. These beverages help to combat acidity in the body.

DID YOU KNOW THAT SEX IS BENEFICIAL.

How-so you ask?

- Helps Keep Your Immune System Humming research and studies show at Wilkes University in Pennsylvania where a survey was conducted that more college students that were highly sexually active had reduce issues of sicknesses so it builds the immune system. So let's get into it ladies.

- Longing for a more lively sex life? "Having sex will make sex better and will improve your libido by itself. anything that you practice you certainly get better at it. That to includes sex. A lot of women suffer with low libido. What is Libido exactly it's the sexual instinct or erotic pleasure or desire. Your libido is otherwise known your 'sex drive'. Libido varies from woman to woman and can be influenced by a range of different factors. Loss or reduction of libido can be experienced at any age and may result in:

reduced desire to have sex. So I know you're asking how is having sex going to increase from having sex if I have low libido" simple fact is I have no desire at all".

SIGNS OF LOW LIBIDO

Low Sex Drive in Women:

- little to no interest in sexual activity.
- few to no sexual thoughts or fantasies.
- disinterest in initiating sex.
- difficulty getting pleasure from sex.
- lack of pleasurable sensations when the genitals are stimulated

HOW TO BOOST YOUR LIBIDO

There are vitamins that are proven to surge your libido

- Vitamin A
- Magnesium
- Vitamin C
- Vitamin B6 & B3
- Vitamin E is actually called the Sex Vitamin for it pumps your nether regions with blood and oxygen, it also regulates your sex hormones so that your libido gets a boost…

There are also drinks that assist with sexual stamina

- Aloe vera juice…
- Pomegranate juice…
- Milk…

- Banana shake...

- Watermelon juice…

Whoa and check this out! Bananas contain the bromelain enzyme that actually increase libido and reverse impotence in men. "How about that" banana lovers. Also, they are potent sources of potassium and B vitamins like riboflavin, which increase the body's overall energy levels.

HOME REMEDIES

- Exercise, Regular aerobic exercise and strength training can increase your stamina, improve your body image, lift your mood and boost your libido. Exercising actually gives you more energy to burn off ladies. So let's get active.

- Stress less…

- Manage Anxiety

- Communicate with your partner…

- Set aside time for intimacy…

- Add a little spice to your sex life…

- Get enough sleep. Sleep is incredibly important for your health — including your sex drive…

- Check your medications

- Practice mindfulness

- Try yoga

- Maintain a healthful weight

- Try herbal remedies

- Focus on foreplay

Lastly the most natural viagra for women is Red Ginseng

- Ginseng — red ginseng in particular — may aid low libido and improve sexual function. In fact, a review of 10 studies found that red ginseng was effective at improving sexual arousal in women with menopause.

SUFFERING WITH VAGINAL DRYNESS

Vaginal dryness is a thing of the past. How to naturally rid yourself of vaginal dryness without the quite so often gynecologist office visits.

LET'S TALK LUBRICATIONS

- Vaginal dryness can have physical or psychological causes
- Vaginal lubrication is often closely tied to levels of the hormone estrogen, which changes at various life stages
- Medications (including hormonal birth control) may cause vaginal dryness
- You can have a happy and healthy sex life even if you don't produce much natural vaginal lubrication

Did you know vaginal dryness can happen at any age. Symptoms may include a burning sensation, vaginal discomfort or itching, abnormal vaginal discharge or pain during sex or there can be a number of reasons for vaginal dryness, both psychological and physiological. Whether you're drier than you would like to be during sexual activity, or are experiencing more general discomfort due to vaginal dryness.

SOME CAUSES

- Vaginal dryness and estrogen levels

The hormone estrogen helps to keep the vagina moist and to maintain the thickness of the vaginal lining. Atrophic vaginitis (vulvovaginal atrophy) is a common condition that can occur when the ovaries produce a decreased amount of estrogen, which includes the prominent symptom of vaginal dryness.

- Your body produces less estrogen.

- At the time of menopause then it is classified as genitourinary syndrome of menopause

- After , particularly if breastfeeding

- Medications which interfere with reproductive hormone regulation, such as those which treat breast cancer or certain gonadotrophin releasing hormone agonists.

- Removal of the ovaries, chemotherapy, or radiation therapy of the pelvis.

If you're noticing dryness during vaginal sex, this could be for a number of reasons. Maybe what your partner is doing just doesn't turn you on. If you feel turned on but are still dry, your body might simply need time to catch up with your brain. If you're noticing vaginal dryness along with a lack of sexual desire, you may be experiencing low libido, which can be caused by a number of factors including medication and health conditions. Or you just might not be all that into your partner or the acts you are performing together.

Your sexual desire is influenced by some of the same hormones that fluctuate with your cycle, like estrogen and progesterone.

You may find your desire tends to increase in the days leading up to ovulation and decrease after ovulation is over. Sex drive may be lower when more progesterone is produced during the luteal phase (the days after ovulation and leading up to menstruation). Exactly how reproductive hormones influence desire and preference isn't the same for everyone; some people report a higher sex drive as part of their premenstrual experience, while other present with decreased libido. Tracking desire throughout your cycle can help you discover what's true for you.

If you're experiencing dryness since being on medication or a form of hormonal birth control: talk to your healthcare provider about trying another one that's a better fit for your body. If you suspect your dryness could be caused by low estrogen levels, there are several treatment options: vaginal moisturizers or lubricants, local vaginal estrogen cream or tablet, systemic estrogen (and progesterone) therapy, or sometimes selective estrogen receptor modulators (SERMs). See your healthcare provider to find out what's the best option for you. If what your sexual partner is doing doesn't work for you: you could try discussing your sexual likes and dislikes—you may even find that just talking about it increases your arousal. If you lack desire for your partner, it's probably time to do some relationship re-evaluation, whether you want to remain in your current relationship or investigate if any health issues could be the cause of your low libido. If you feel turned on but you're not wet: spending more time on foreplay can be one way to increase your natural lubrication. Another option is to use personal lubricant (lube) during sexual activity or masturbation.

Lubricants made with water or silicone can be used with latex condoms and diaphragms. Oil-based products, such as petroleum jelly, baby oil, mineral oil, or vegetable oils are not healthy to use internally, and are likely to damage latex condoms and/or diaphragms and make them less effective at preventing pregnancy or STIs.

A study published in the journal Obstetrics and Gynecology found that women who had used petroleum jelly as lube in the past month were more than twice as likely as non-users to have bacteria vaginosis Hand or body lotions are not recommended either, as they can be irritating to vaginal tissues.

If you prefer to use something natural, please by all means avoid using food products like olive oil or coconut oil as this can lead to yeast infections or bacterial vaginosis. Instead, try an organic lubricant or a water-based lube without additives.

Other possible reasons of vaginal dryness are.

Aside from sexual arousal and estrogen levels, there are additional factors that can affect vaginal lubrication:

- Vaginal dryness can be a side effect of some medications and contraceptives. Talk to your healthcare provider to find out if the source of your vaginal dryness could actually be your medication or contraception. Cigarette smokers have been shown to have an increased risk of an earlier menopause transition as compared to non smokers. This means that atrophic vaginitis symptoms may appear at a younger age in this population. Sjögren's syndrome could be another cause of possible vaginal (and other symptoms of dryness). This is an autoimmune disease where the body's glands aren't able to produce enough moisture.

If you've checked out everything else and still don't find the culprit, you might have an allergy to chemicals in soap, detergent, lubricant or hygiene products—these can also cause vaginal dryness or irritation. Try switching to natural products and wash with unperfumed soap or just water, and see if your symptoms improve.

Research has linked the practice of douching with increased risk of bacterial and yeast infections, pelvic inflammatory disease, cervical cancer, increased transmission of STIs, upper genital tract infections, endometritis (inflammation of the lining of the uterus), and other adverse health outcomes. Lastly for a all natural approach for vaginal dryness, use Yoni Steaming it will certainly assist by creating blood flow to the vagina which causes natural secretions.

GOODBYE BLADDER LEAKAGE

OVERACTIVE BLADDER

OAB affects how your bladder stores urine: your brain signals your bladder to empty, even when it isn't full. This may cause your bladder muscles to contract. These frequent or uncontrollable contractions can lead to symptoms of OAB, which are urgency, frequency, and leakage.

If you have these symptoms, you're not alone. As many as 46 million Americans 40 years of age or older have reported symptoms of OAB. According to the American Urological Association, OAB:

- occurs in both men and women
- may affect your daily activities due to lack of bladder control
- can cause embarrassment, leading some
- to just learn to cope with the condition

Are you planning your daily activities around being close to bathrooms to avoid urine leaks and accidents? It may be time to have an honest talk with your healthcare professional (HCP). Lifestyle changes can help.

A healthy bladder muscle expands as it fills with urine. Once it's about half full, nerves in the bladder tell you it's time to urinate.

OAB interrupts the normal storage of urine. It causes the bladder muscle to suddenly contract before the bladder is full.

This can lead to frequent and sudden, strong urges to urinate, sometimes with leakage.

The symptoms of OAB can have you searching for a bathroom, anytime, anywhere. They can come over you suddenly, and they are hard to control.

Feeling the Urgency which is when you feel a strong need to urinate that is hard to control. It may even be strong enough to cause urine leakage.

Frequency is the need to urinate too often. Urinating more than seven times during waking hours is one of the primary symptoms of OAB.

Bladder leakage, is when you accidentally urinate after a sudden, uncontrollable urge. Some people cope with leakage by wearing absorbent products, like pads, in case of accidents.

Or could it be urinary incontinence.? Loss of bladder control, varying from a slight loss of urine after sneezing, coughing, or laughing to complete inability to control urination.

Urinary incontinence can have causes that aren't due to underlying disease. Examples include intoxication, unavailability of bathrooms, coughing, sneezing, extreme anxiety, or intense laughter.

URINARY INCONTINENCE

Can be self treated by,

Doing pelvic floor exercises, avoiding caffeine, and wearing absorbent undergarments may help reduce urinary incontinence. Bladder retraining that involves gradually increasing time until urination may also help.

For many people with urinary incontinence, the following self-help tips and lifestyle changes are enough to relieve symptoms.

- Do daily pelvic floor exercises. ...
- Stop smoking. ...
- Do exercises safely and properly...
- Avoid overly heavy lifting....
- Lose as much excess weight as possible...
- Treat constipation promptly. ...
- Cut down on caffeine. ...
- Cut down on alcohol.

Urinary Incontinence almost never goes away on it's on. But those are a few steps you can take to help relieve your symptoms. "Alleviating urinary incontinence starts with first understanding which type of incontinence you're experiencing and what's causing it.

Urinary incontinence occurs more often in women than in men. Pregnancy childbirth and menopause may contribute to urinary incontinence in women. Weak bladder muscles, overactive bladder muscles, and nerve damage may also cause urinary incontinence in women. Urinary incontinence in women is common and treatable.

Types of urinary incontinence include:

- Stress incontinence.

Urine leaks when you exert pressure on your bladder by coughing, sneezing, laughing, exercising or lifting something heavy.

- Urge incontinence.

- Overflow incontinence. Functional incontinence.

- Mixed incontinence.

Is Urinary Incontinence normal with aging process? One simple answer Yes! However you can assist yourself with the remedies mentioned earlier on. While aging may be a factor, urinary incontinence is not an inevitable part of aging. As shown by this poll, urinary incontinence affects nearly half of women age 50–80.

Let your vagina breathe!

Did you know that sleeping with panties is a total thing of the past.

The older we get the wiser we get, in the history of women, they would sleep in bloomers or ruffle undies at night, not sure why, but whatever the reason was at that point and time, it's a total thing of the past. Nowadays we have the sexiest most inviting sensual sex appeal panties ever, yet we should not wear them for long periods of time. So let's just say for convenience of time, the best time to take a panty break is at night. So feel free ladies to tempt and tease your mate with those sexy under garments, but after all the tempting and teasing is done and over, leave them on the floor for the night. Wearing tight~fitting clothing or pajamas or even underwear can lead to moisture buildup, wearing underwear keeps moisture close to the genital area. This actually allows bacteria and yeast to grow, which can cause infection and other problems. Sleeping freely releases toxins from the body. Also going commando for men helps with a healthy sperm count. And for all ladies who endures the pleasure of a monthly cycle and chooses to wear pads and not tampons, please be sure to use feminine wipes or wash your vagina periodically throughout the day, with changing your menstrual pad whenever it becomes soiled your pad should never be worn all day or overly soaked.

Tampons should be changed often as well. For women who uses tampons it is highly suggested that you wear tampons that come in sizes to choose the tampon that is best fit for your body type. If your tampon is worn too long of a period of time, you put yourself at risk for toxic shock syndrome, or even worst a overgrowth of bacteria called staphylococcus aureus, or short term staph infection. Changing your super or plus tampon at least every six hours reduces your likelihood of developing TSS. Yes you can shower and even bathe with your tampon inserted. It should be absolutely no discomfort at all, if it is either your tampon should be changed immediately due to being to full or either it's not positioned properly. Which it could very well be you did not push it up far enough into the vaginal canal, it's a quick fix, just gently take your middle finger which is your longest finger for most, simply squat and insert your longest finger and push it in just a tad bit more, if you feel pain or simply can not find comfort with using this product, perhaps you should stick to menstrual pads. It is highly suggested if at all possible that is you must wear feminine pads or tampons please use all natural organic items, or use a menstrual cup.

A MENSTRUAL CUP

a menstrual cup is a flexible cup that fits inside your vagina it does not absorb the blood flow as tampons and pads do, the cup actually is a cup specifically designed to fit inside the cavity of the vagina to collect the period flow, as well whenever using this product please boil it first for roughly between 5-10 minutes prior to use. Also whenever using any product/s or prior to touching yourself especially internally wash your hands throughly with mild soap and warm water for at least a minute and rinse throughly. A menstrual cup comes in different sizes and a variety of colors. The sizes are pretty much age and body type selected. If you've never used a menstrual cup before and would like to try it before your cycle, great. Please speak with your gynecologist or certified yoni practitioner about sizing and proper use and to check and see if you're a good candidate for the product.

REASONS WHY SEX HURTS

Wanting sex craving sex but dreading having sex..

Did you know that sex can be painful due to hormone levels. The word that most women dread and wish they could run and hide from is menopause, and menopause after years and years of study and research can now be just another life adjustment. We no longer have to be afraid of the aging process with all the new natural and organic discoveries which have been around for centuries but are new to most of us.

If you are a woman going through the changes of life and find yourself suffering with night sweat, vaginal dryness and painful sex, I need you to know I'm here to help, first off what's going is the elasticity of your vaginal walls have begun to lose stretch and give and this is why you feel the tenderness and or soreness feeling you get during intercourse. Which makes sex quite painful, also as we age the vaginal walls begin to thin out and due to lack of hormones we tend to become less lubricated as we once were. Listen ladies younger and seasoned, every woman will at some point in life deal with the issue of menopause. And I'm here to tell you a few things that works to help aid and support the trying issues of menopause, but first off there are also other medical issues that can be the cause of painful sex such as an infection called thrush for men or a sexual transmitted disease (STI) such as genital herpes, chlamydia, gonorrhoea for both men and women.

Also lack of sexual arousal at any age, or vaginismus, which is a condition where the muscles in or around the vagina shuts tightly, making sex painful or impossible. Genital irritation or allergy caused by spermicides latex condoms or products such as shampoos or soaps. Pains felt inside the pelvis can be caused by conditions such as pelvic inflammatory disease(PID)

- endometriosis
- fibroids growing near your vagina or cervix
- Irritable bowel syndrome (IBS)
- constipation

Painful sex in men include:

- Infections like thrush, which can cause soreness and itching and some STI's, such as herpes
- a tight foreskin, which can make penetration painful, as the for skin is pushed back.
- small tears in the foreskin that can't be seen but causes soreness and a sharp, stinging pain around the tear
- Inflammation of the prostate gland (prostatitis)
- testicle pain and swelling which can sometimes be caused by getting sexually aroused but not ejaculating (coming) it can also be a sign of an infection, such as chlamydia.

If you are a male and have or experiencing any of these complications please speak with your GP Doctor or a health care professional immediately. They'll try to find the cause of the problem and be able to tell you what treatment best fits you.

For example if have pain, unusual discharge, itchiness or soreness around your genitals they may recommend treatment for thrush or an STI test.

If your vagina is dry, you may be advised to try using a lubricant just remember to use a water based product, if you're using condoms because oil based lubricants can damage them and make them ineffective.

If you have an allergy or an irritation around your genitals, you may be advised to avoid using products that could be causing it.

If there's an emotional reason or anxiety that's causing problems, a counselor or sex therapist may be able to help- your GP or sexual health clinic can refer you to one

But for all those who are in search of a all natural approach after seeing MD, Gynecologist or GP Doctor whichever you prefer, to help aid with the issues of a reoccurrence of symptoms. Try speaking with a Certified trained Yoni Practitioner, Yoni And Joni steaming has been around for centuries but in most recent years have become popular. Yoni steaming can most certainly help with reoccurring yeast infection and bacteria vaginosis,it also helps with menopausal symptoms such as, hot flashes and night sweats. Yoni steaming can also assist with vaginal dryness or your Gynecologist can also prescribe a vaginal hormonal cream to help aid with painful sex which it also overtime helps with the elasticity of the vaginal walls or you can purchase OTC organic natural lubricants to aid in more pleasurable sexual encounters. Yoni steaming helps with fibroids and cyst by breaking them down and causing them to decrease in a shrinking size making them passable through the vaginal cavity. Yoni steaming helps assist with pelvic floor support, along with kegel exercises. Yoni steaming keeps your PH balanced and your vagina healthy, riding all toxins, old blood, dead tissue and removes old semen from your womb.

Joni steaming helps men with bloating, releasing toxins from the body, increasing sperm count and as well maintaining a healthy prostate life, reducing the swelling in the prostate which causes frequent urination as well as the uncontrollable urgency of urination during the night, which causes lack of rest. Joni steaming helps with penile dysfunction as well as creating a amazing circulation of blood flow which causes a all natural arousal effect.

 Before trying either Yoni V Steaming or Joni Steaming please check with a certified Yoni Practitioner and find out if you're a good candidate for the all natural practice.

SEX IS THERAPEUTIC

I know it may seem unrealistic, but studies suggest that sex therapy may actual help people with a history of sexual trauma. With a combination of trauma based therapy with sex positive techniques may be more promising and effective than just trauma based therapy alone. First off let's dabble into this with a complete understanding that any form of abuse is not ok in any form or fashion, that trauma is established and birthed by hurt, affliction or pain caused by another.

With all victims of a crime it is highly suggested that you seek professional therapy immediately, to help navigate and process the act of violence that you have recently encountered and have had to endure, accept the fact that you are a survivor and you have every right to that title.

But for people who are simply just over worked, stressed out or in need of a natural relaxant, I need for you to know that sex is therapeutic, there is such a thing called tantric sex, I know you thought I was going in another direction, but for today this is our angle, it's not for the end result of orgasm, but when speaking of Tantric sex we are talking about a slow mind blowing meditative sex, simply enjoying the state of mind that takes a sexual sensual journey and sensations of your body, what happens is you move sexual energy throughout your body for healing and enlightenment.

First off the word Tantric means woven together, you do not have to practice Hindu or Buddhist to practice tantric sex, but they surely do, the practice brings together the spirituality and the sexuality and emphasizes the importance of intimacy during sexual encounters. Most successful marriages and unions practice tantric sex rather they even know it, when in the act of making love to one's mate such as you husband or wife and you feel such a deep connection, a force, a power sort to speak, a surge of power of some sort, as if you two are completely as one and they are an extension of yourself, if you've ever experienced that type connection with your significant other you have a tantric marriage. Where there is no need for actual intercourse sometimes, because you're so connected and powered by the touch of your mates hand or just them being close to you. It's totally mind blowing, and if you have a tantric relationship lucky you, and if you haven't experienced a love on that level yet, keep looking.

When overworked, stressed or just drained, sex with your mate can actually be a natural relaxant. If you can then set the mood for a steaming passion filled night, but if no adequate time for mood setting and you need a quick release of tension by all means, make it count, deep shallow breaths, making sure your body is not tensed and let your mind focus on warm island beach waters that gently brushes against your body causing a build up of emotions all while in your mind you hear the island birds and the palms rustling softly. I guarantee you thee most satisfying pleasure ever.

When thinking of sex, some tend to think it's a dirty word, it truly is not and it should be educated more and talked about more often and have a better understanding of it and responsibility of those who partake in the act itself. That would eliminate more STD's and unwanted pregnancies. Consensual sex is healthy and should be pleasurable without agony, pain or force, if you are not experiencing the proper love, support and affection, that just may cause you to not enjoy sex as you should.

When it comes to your body and you're unsure, it feels wrong or it's just a sense of uncertainty, seek medical attention, it's always better to know than to assume.

NUTRIENTS FOR BETTER LIBIDO AND LUBRICATION

Did you know there are some foods that are packed with awesome nutrients that's helps perk up your libido

One which is my ultimate favorite, but not so much by others oysters, most everyone has heard about the aphrodisiac properties in oysters.

- Salmon
- Nuts and seeds
- Apples

- Beets

- Red wines

- Some meats

- A nutritious diet can benefit your sex life in many ways.

- Boosting your libido

- Improving blood flow

IMPROVING YOUR STAMINA

As we've stated earlier on menopause certainly plays a major part in vaginal dryness due to hormonal issues. But there are also other issues as we've stated that can also cause vaginal dryness, but here are some supplements that can assist with that issue, vitamin E and D, sea buckthorn oil, hyaluronic acid, my favorite fish oil.

Natural lubricants also are jojoba coconut oil, aloe vera, vitamin E suppositories which stimulates the vagina.

 Eating a diet rich in vegetables and lean proteins and low in foods that contains sugar and saturated fats, can also help to prevent disorders that can effect your libido like metabolic syndrome and hor monal conditions. When looking for meats look for meats high in carnitine arginine and zinc.

Smooth blood flow is crucial to all sexual response in male and female.

Foods are certainly a major factor in how good your sex life can be, while certain foods can spike your libido and boost your arousal casing your energy to last longer in bed, other foods can totally do the complete opposite and cause your energy to be very low or non existent all together.

FOODS FOR FERTILITY

If trying to conceive or wanting to improve your reproductive health in general, there are certain foods you should certainly avoid. And certain ones you must include in your diet, cash in on foods that contain folic acid and vitamin C these nutrients are important to avoid birth defects in your child and strengthen organs. Broccoli, beetroot, lentils, oranges, tomatoes,are also good choices. And unfortunately steer clear of fish ice cream meat and alcohol

SPERM HEALTH

Always think zinc when thinking of your sperm count or sperm health, zinc really helps with sperm production, so eat plenty almonds, sesame seeds, leafy green vegetables and brown rice to add more zinc to your body. Foods enriched with vitamin E is also very beneficial, also add foods with Omega 3 to help improve blood circulation and neurological connections with your testicles.

WHAT IS THAT SMELL?

The root of vaginal odor

Ladies I know you've heard before you smell it before anyone else does, so if you smell it please believe if not already they soon will. Now what is the cause of vaginal odor and how can you rid yourself of it.? Bacteria vaginosis is known for its fishy foul odor, which is also the most common vaginal odor. Then there is trichomoniasis a (STI) sexual transmitted infection. Rectovaginal fistula; a rare condition in which an opening between the rectum and the vagina allows feces to leak into the vagina. Vaginal cancer symptoms include heavy vaginal discharge, that can have a strong odor. Cervical cancer symptoms can include a strong (bad smelling) discharge, cancer is a rare cause of abnormal vaginal odor.

However, temporary vaginal odor is common, and can and sometimes do resolve on its on, in this case it can be due to diet, foods with a strong odor such as garlic or fish can cause odor changes in the vagina. In order to determine which type of bacteria that may be causing your vaginitis, your doctor will take a sample of discharge. The most common cause of abnormal vaginal odor is high levels of Gardnerella bacteria.

Abnormal vaginal odor goes away without treatment at least a third of the time. If it does not resolve on its own, your healthcare provider will prescribe antibiotics. These can be taken in a pill or cream form. However after you've seen and been treated by you primary care physician or your gynecologist, be sure to look into the all natural approach of Yoni steaming by a trained certified Yoni practitioner to assist with reoccurrence of vaginal odor. As well practicing good hygiene by bathing and showering regularly helps. Avoidance of douching which is an intravaginal liquid cleansing solution. Douching can upset PH levels in the vagina and lead to an infection.

Women who have multiple sex partners and does not use a condom can also cause themselves to have a vaginal odor, from the mixture of blood and semen and multiple diets alongside with other health factors to be considered. This is a quick way to get and transmit a sexual transmitted disease but also throw off your ph balance. With STD women are proven to know a lot sooner than most men, due to women early onset of itching, burning, discharge and irritation. If you have any of the following signs or issues please see your primary care physician or gynecologist right away. If you have any of those signs or issues please see your primary care physician or gynecologist right away.

HEALTH LITERACY IS VITAL.

This book is to educate you and give insight on womb care aka "Cookie" care and the awesome centuries old treasured benefits of herbs in combination of steaming with herbs and how you too can benefit from it.

Joni steaming for men is solely used in practice of promoting healthy prostate life.